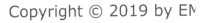

Table of Contents

INTRODUCTION

The study of adolescents found that, irrespective of gender, adolescents with ADHD had nearly double the number of lifetime sexual partners. That finding is consistent with Barkley's follow-up study of ADHD children. He and his colleagues found that ADHD predicted early sexual activity and early parenthood. Similar findings were reported by Flory and colleagues in retrospective study of young adults. Childhood ADHD predicted earlier initiation of sexual activity and intercourse, more sexual partners, more casual sex, and more partner pregnancies. When my colleagues and I studied 1001 adults in the community, we found that adults with ADHD endorsed less stability in their love relationships, felt less able to provide emotional support to their loved ones, experienced more sexual dysfunction and had higher divorce rates. The research literature about love, sex and ADHD is small, but it is consistent. there is an increasing awareness that attention deficit hyperactivity disorder (ADHD) is present in adults and that the symptoms and functional consequences of the disorder have been ongoing since childhood. The core symptoms of ADHD include inattention, distractibility, hyperactivity, and impulsivity. Although the hyperactivity symptoms may abate in some ADHD adults, the inattention and distractibility symptoms often persist and contribute to interpersonal, social, family, academic, and work-related difficulties. In contrast to children and adolescents, adult ADHD has been less diagnosed and is often mis-diagnosed, under-treated when recognized, or not treated at all. Consequently, this book explores the impact of ADHD on a couple's sex life and relationship. It explains how a better sex life will benefit your relationship (and vice versa) and why that's especially important for couples with one partner with ADHD. Written in a readable and entertaining style, ADHD After Dark offers clear information on sexuality and relationships and is full of valuable advice on how to improve both. This guide will be an essential read for adults with ADHD, as well as their partners or spouses, and therapists who work with ADHD clients and couples.

What is ADHD

Attention deficit hyperactivity disorder (ADHD) is a mental health disorder that can cause above-normal levels of hyperactive and impulsive behaviors. People with ADHD may also have trouble focusing their attention on a single task or sitting still for long periods of time. Both adults and children can have ADHD. It's a diagnosis the American Psychiatric Association (APA) recognizes. Learn about types of ADHD and symptoms in both children and adults.

ADHD symptoms

A wide range of behaviors are associated with ADHD. Some of the more common ones include:

• having trouble focusing or concentrating on tasks

• being forgetful about completing tasks

• being easily distracted

• having difficulty sitting still

• interrupting people while they're talking

If you or your child has ADHD, you may have some or all of these symptoms. The symptoms you have depend on the type of ADHD you have. Explore a list of ADHD symptoms common in children.

Types of ADHD

To make ADHD diagnoses more consistent, the APA has grouped the condition into three categories, or types. These types are predominantly inattentive, predominantly hyperactivity-impulsive, and a combination of both.

Predominantly inattentive

As the name suggests, people with this type of ADHD have extreme difficulty focusing, finishing tasks, and following instructions.

Experts also think that many children with the inattentive type of ADHD may not receive a proper diagnosis because they don't tend to disrupt the classroom. This type is most common among girls with ADHD.

Predominantly hyperactive-impulsive type

People with this type of ADHD show primarily hyperactive and impulsive behavior. This can include fidgeting, interrupting people while they're talking, and not being able to wait their turn. Although inattention is less of a concern with this type of ADHD, people with predominantly hyperactive-impulsive ADHD may still find it difficult to focus on tasks.

Combined hyperactive-impulsive and inattentive type

This is the most common type of ADHD. People with this combined type of ADHD display both inattentive and hyperactive symptoms. These include an inability to pay attention, a tendency toward impulsiveness, and above-normal levels of activity and energy.

The type of ADHD you or your child has will determine how it's treated. The type you have can change over time, so your treatment may change, too. Learn more about the three types of ADHD.

ADD vs. ADHD

You may have heard the terms "ADD" and "ADHD" and wondered what the difference is between them.

ADD, or attention deficit disorder, is an outdated term. It was previously used to describe people who have problems paying attention but aren't hyperactive. The type of ADHD called predominantly inattentive is now used in place of ADD.

ADHD is the current overarching name of the condition. The term ADHD became official in May 2013, when the APA released the Diagnostic and Statistical Manual of Mental Disorders, Fifth Edition (DSM-5). This manual is what doctors refer to when making diagnoses for mental health conditions. Get a better understanding of the difference between ADD and ADHD.

Adult ADHD

More than 60 percent Trusted Source of children with ADHD still exhibit symptoms as adults. But for many people, ADHD symptoms decrease or become less frequent as they get older.

That said, treatment is important. Untreated ADHD in adults can have a negative impact on many aspects of life. Symptoms such as trouble managing time, forgetfulness, and impatience can cause problems at work, home, and in all types of relationships. Find out more about the signs and symptoms of ADHD in adults and how they can impact your life.

What causes ADHD

Despite how common ADHD is, doctors and researchers still aren't sure what causes the condition. It's believed to have neurological origins. Genetics may also play a role. ResearchTrusted Source suggests that a reduction in dopamine is a factor in ADHD. Dopamine is a chemical in the brain that helps move signals from one nerve to another. It plays a role in triggering emotional responses and movements. Other researchTrusted Source suggests a structural difference in the brain. Findings indicate that people with ADHD have less gray matter volume. Gray matter includes the brain areas that help with:

• speech

• self-control

• decision-making

• muscle control

Researchers are still studying potential causes of ADHD, such as smoking during pregnancy. Find out more about the potential causes and risk factors of ADHD.

ADHD testing and diagnosis

There's no single test that can tell if you or your child has ADHD. A recent studyTrusted Source highlighted the benefits of a new test to diagnose adult ADHD, but many clinicians believe an ADHD diagnosis can't be made based on one test.

To make a diagnosis, your doctor will assess any symptoms you or your child has had over the previous six months. Your doctor will likely gather information from teachers or family members and may use checklists and rating scales to review symptoms. They'll also do a physical exam to check for other health problems. Learn more about ADHD rating scales and what they can and cannot do.

If you suspect that you or your child has ADHD, talk to your doctor about getting an evaluation. For your child, you can also talk to their school counselor. Schools regularly assess children for problems that may be affecting their educational performance.

For the assessment, provide your doctor or counselor with notes and observations about you or your child's behavior.

If they suspect ADHD, they may refer you or your child to an ADHD specialist. Depending on the diagnosis, they may also suggest making an appointment with a psychiatrist or neurologist.

ADHD treatment

Treatment for ADHD typically includes behavioral therapies, medication, or both.

Types of therapy include psychotherapy, or talk therapy. With talk therapy, you or your child will discuss how ADHD affects your life and ways to help you manage it. Another therapy type is behavioral therapy. This therapy can help you or your child with learning how to monitor and manage your behavior.

Medication can also be very helpful when you're living with ADHD. ADHD medications are designed to affect brain chemicals in a way that enables you to better control your impulses and actions.

ADHD medication

The two main types of medications used to treat ADHD are stimulants and nonstimulants.

Central nervous system (CNS) stimulants are the most commonly prescribed ADHD medications. These drugs work by increasing the amounts of the brain chemicals dopamine and norepinephrine.

Examples of these drugs include methylphenidate (Ritalin) and amphetamine-based stimulants (Adderall).

If stimulants don't work well for you or your child, or if they cause troublesome side effects, your doctor may suggest a nonstimulant medication. Certain nonstimulant medications work by increasing levels of norepinephrine in the brain.

These medications include atomoxetine (Strattera) and some antidepressants such as bupropion (Wellbutrin).

ADHD medications can have many benefits, as well as side effects. Learn more about medication options for adults with ADHD.

Natural remedies for ADHD

In addition to or instead of medication, several remedies have been suggested to help improve ADHD symptoms.

For starters, following a healthy lifestyle may help you or your child manage ADHD symptoms. The Centers for

Disease Control and Prevention (CDC)Trusted Source recommends the following:

• eat a healthy, balanced diet

• get at least 60 minutes of physical activity per day

• get plenty of sleep

• limit daily screen time from phones, computers, and TV

Studies have also shown that yoga Trusted Source, tai chi, and spending time outdoors can help calm overactive minds and may ease ADHD symptoms. Mindfulness meditation is another option. ResearchTrusted Source in adults and teens has shown meditation to have positive effects on attention and thought processes, as well as on anxiety and depression.

Avoiding certain allergens and food additives are also potential ways to help reduce ADHD symptoms. Learn more about these and other nondrug approaches to addressing ADHD.

ADHD and Sex

Helping people with ADHD improve sexual connection and communication

People with ADHD tend to have more sex issues than those without ADHD difficulty focusing during sex, an increased rate of risky sexual behaviors, and a need for sexual novelty. Ari Tuckman Psy.D., MBA, a psychologist, ADHD specialist, and author of three books on ADHD, including More Attention, Less Deficit: Success Strategies for Adults with ADHD, tells us more about how ADHD impacts sex lives—and what to do about it.

What are some of the most common issues people with ADHD face in regards to sex

People in happy relationships tend to have more sex, but ADHD (especially when undiagnosed and untreated) can negatively impact a couple's happiness. It's hard to feel sexually attracted to and generous with someone that you are angry at. It's also possible that sex just gets squeezed out of the day because one or both partners run out of time or energy.

How often do people with ADHD experience difficulties or stress related to sex

People with ADHD have the same difficulties with sex as people without ADHD, but perhaps more often or more intensely. I call this the ADHD multiplier: the ADHD multiplies the difficulties, but doesn't really create unique problems that others aren't also experiencing. Many of the sexual problems for these folks isn't about sex per se, but about the relationship struggles that undermine a satisfying sex life.

How common of an issue is sex addiction, including porn addiction, in ADHD

There is some debate as to whether one can actually be addicted to sex or porn, but what is clear is that people with ADHD tend to have more difficulties with problematic sexual behavior. This can include making impulsive sexual choices, with all the consequences that that can bring. People who are thrill-seekers (such as some people with the hyperactive and impulsive symptoms of ADHD) are more likely to engage in problematic sexual behaviors, including over-using pornography.

What treatments do you recommend for a person with ADHD whose high sex drive has lead to difficulties in their current relationship? Is individual therapy or couples therapy recommended? Depending on the severity of the situation, it would probably be helpful to engage in both couples and individual therapy, for both partners. I would first want to address the ADHD, probably with medication, and be sure that there are no other conditions here, such as bipolar disorder. I would also want to explore with the client what is driving that high sex drive. For some it's simply that they have a biologically higher sex drive. If this is the case, I would want to work with the couple to help them decide how this is to be handled in the relationship, what kinds of sexual behaviors are acceptable or not, etc. The couple needs to negotiate this out and find a solution that works for both partners. However, if some of that high sex drive comes from the person's attempts to self-medicate and feel better, for example when bored or frustrated, then I would want to work with that client on more effective ways of dealing with uncomfortable feelings and situations.

How often does distraction play into sexual difficulties for people with ADHD, such as difficulty achieving orgasm

Everybody gets distracted during sex sometimes, but people with ADHD may be more likely. Losing focus during sex can cause men to lose some or all of their erection or for women to lose some of their lubrication and can delay orgasm for both. The important thing, for

17

both partners, is to not make too much out of the distraction or take it too personally. Simply refocus and get back in the game!

Why is novelty, especially sexual novelty, is such a turn-on for the ADHD brain

People with ADHD will often get bored more easily than others or will more quickly get used to something. Therefore they will seek novelty to re-engage their attention and cause their brain to light up again. Just as it can happen in the classroom, it can also happen in the bedroom. This doesn't necessarily mean that a couple's sex life needs to get forever more intense, but it may be that the couple will need a bigger repertoire of activities, positions, and/or locations that they rotate through in order to keep both partners interested.

A 2010 study by Garcia et al. that found that people with ADHD may be more likely to cheat. What are the factors that you feel may contribute to this increased rate of cheating?

Some of this is probably due to the person with ADHD making an impulsive decision in the moment without a clear intent ahead of time. For example, kissing someone in a bar. However, people in unhappy relationships are more likely to engage in extramarital activities and ADHD (especially when undiagnosed and untreated) can lead to more unhappiness. So sometimes affairs are a way to cope with an unhappy relationship, even though it will often make a bad situation worse.

According to Barkley et al. (2008), people with ADHD are more likely to have sexually transmitted diseases and have more sexual partners. What are some ways that people with ADHD can protect themselves?

I suspect that this is mostly the result of impulsive decision making regarding sexual partners and activities. Also, it often takes some planning and delay of gratification in the moment to practice safe sex. If you struggle with that, you are more likely to have unprotected sex. If you're someone who sometimes engages in unplanned sex, especially with people with unknown STD status, it is important to always have condoms with you--and then to really make a point of using them. It's probably also a good idea to avoid drinking too much or doing too many drugs in certain situations that are more likely to lead to unplanned sex. You may even want to avoid certain situations entirely, because it's too easy to fall into behaviors that you will later regret. Finally, you may find that medication helps you slow down and make better thought out decisions.

Because people with ADHD may have difficulty expressing their sexual concerns or needs to their partner, what are some ways these topics can be addressed?

As in any other relationship, it's important to be able to talk openly and honestly about sexual desires and concerns. However, in order to be able to have good conversations in bed, you have to be having good conversations outside of bed too--and not just about sex, but about all the other parts of the relationship. The better you address the other matters in the relationship, the more generous your partner will be sexually and also the stronger position you are in when discussing sexual matters. If there are too many other unresolved issues in the relationship, your partner isn't likely to be sexually receptive.

There are many ways that attention deficit hyperactivity disorder (ADHD) can affect your sex life. If you live with ADHD, you might notice that you are hypersensitive to sensory stimulation, making sensual touch feel irritating and even annoying. Or perhaps your level of sexual desire changes drastically from one day to the next.

On the flip side, some people with ADHD have such a high sex drive and need for stimulation and novelty, such as pornography, that it causes problems in a partnership.

People with ADHD may also be prone to sexual risk-taking such as unprotected sex or having multiple sex partners. The disorder is associated with a drop in neurotransmitters, which may lead to these types of impulsive behaviors.

There's even something called post-orgasm irritability that can happen with ADHD, where the drop in dopamine following intense pleasure leads to feelings of sadness and depression.

If Your Partner Has ADHD

As the partner of someone living with this disorder, you might notice that your partner becomes distracted during intercourse and easily loses focus and interest, which you might interpret as rejection. It's important to understand that ADHD causes trouble concentrating in many areas of life, and sex is often no exception—and it usually has nothing to do with the person's interest in their partner.

Let's not forget the exaggerated feelings that someone with ADHD may experience, such as anger and frustration, can create feelings of conflict in any romantic relationship, and this conflict can result in difficulties connecting sexually as well.

ADHD AND SEX

First and foremost, it's crucial to take ADHD medications as prescribed, and the good news is, many of them don't lower sex drive or sexual desire. In fact, because they increase your ability to focus, they may actually improve your sex life. However, antidepressants are sometimes prescribed for ADHD, and they can indeed lower sex drive. If that is a significant issue or concern, bring it up with your physician. You may be able to lower the dose or switch medications. Beyond that, there are several steps you can take to overcome your challenges from ADHD in the bedroom.

Communication is key. If your ADHD is causing sexual issues, tell your partner that your distraction or other ADHD-driven behaviors are not his or her fault and not a reflection of your level of desire and attraction. Share what you like and what bothers you during foreplay and sex. If you don't like certain smells or lighting, set up your environment in a way that is more comfortable for you. If you don't enjoy certain positions or types of sex, tell your partner what you prefer. If your partner has ADHD, encourage him or her to openly share with you and listen without judgment.

Get rid of distractions. Since it can be hard enough to stay engaged during intercourse, eliminate anything around you that might cause you to lose focus, such as the television. You might also practice releasing the stresses of the day through meditation, yoga, or journaling before getting under the sheets with your partner, to get ahead of any worries on your mind.

Seek the health of a qualified sex therapist or mental health professional. Many couples dealing with ADHD benefit from talk therapy and counseling to improve their sex lives. It helps open lines of communication and bring clarity to misunderstandings and arguments, leading to more intimacy and by extension, better sex.

ADHD IN MARRIAGE

Getting married usually means you have a partner in life. Someone to share the ups and downs of life with, including parenthood, running the household and providing each other with emotional support.

However, if your partner has ADHD, the partnership can become lopsided as you find you are taking care of your partner's responsibilities as well as your own. As the non-ADHD spouse, you may feel you don't have a partner, but instead have someone to corral, organize and direct like a child.

It is easy to see why non-ADHD spouses begin to feel isolated, distant, overwhelmed, resentful, angry, critical and accusatory while the ADHD spouse can feel nagged at, rejected and stressed. When frustrations and tempers become more difficult to control, the marriage may begin to unravel.

Often neither partner realizes that ADHD is the cause of these problems. Dr. David W. Goodman, M.D., assistant professor of Psychiatry and Behavioral Sciences at the Johns Hopkins University School of Medicine and Director of the Adult Attention Deficit Disorder Center of Maryland, says "Many adults incorrectly assume or have inaccurately been told that an individual cannot have ADHD as an adult. This is simply not true."

Dr. Goodman also explains that ADHD is highly genetic. For some adults, a diagnosis is made after their own children are evaluated and diagnosed with ADHD. As the parents learn more and more about ADHD, they may begin to recognize the ADHD traits in themselves.

Adult symptoms of ADHD are similar to childhood symptoms with inattention, distractibility, taking longer to get things done, problems with time management, scatteredness, forgetfulness, and procrastination. They don't develop in adulthood, rather they persist into adulthood. Symptoms also tend to escalate as an individual's environment becomes more stressed and as demands in life increase. It can be a huge relief to finally understand and put a name to the condition causing the problems.

Treatment Issues

"If the ADHD spouse is receptive to diagnosis and treatment, functionality typically improves fairly dramatically," notes Dr. Goodman. Treatment is not only critical; it is often a real eye opener for individuals. Not all adults with ADHD are open to treatment, which can be frustrating for their spouse who sees treatment as a way for their relationship to improve.

"The larger challenge for the non-ADHD spouse," says Dr. Goodman "is when their partner has never received evaluation or treatment, is prejudiced against psychiatry, or has had no exposure to psychiatry and is reluctant or afraid of being labeled, or afraid of having to take medication."

If these are adults with children who are receiving treatment for ADHD, sometimes the dramatic improvements seen in their child has an effect on the ADHD adult's perceptions. Most people want to get better and improve their functioning. When they see their child is functioning so much better with treatment, the adult begins to wonder whether they couldn't do better, too.

When Dr. Goodman encounters reluctant patients, he takes a "let's just sit down and talk" approach. If medicine is indicated, he encourages patients to try it for a month or two. At the end of that period, if the individual is not seeing any improvements or doesn't like how he or she is functioning, the individual can choose to simply discontinue the medicine.

This approach gives the patient a better feeling of control over treatment. For some individuals, there is anxiety or worry about losing control. In order to maintain that control, they may resist treatment. "People want to feel in control of their psychiatric treatment, especially in regards to how it affects their mental functioning," explains Dr. Goodman who typically first provides education and accurate information about adult ADHD and works hard to make an in-road and engage reluctant patients.

Treatment is a partnership with the doctor, but the ultimate control is held by the patient. "Most people understand that when they come into treatment they are functioning 'less than'," says Dr. Goodman. Generally, people want to get better. If they are able to experience the improved quality of life resulting from treatment, most individuals become invested in continuing. "Few people chose to function at a lower level once they experience the benefits."

Advice for the Partner

Dr. Goodman says it is very helpful for the non-ADHD spouse to develop an understanding of the impact ADHD can have on an individual's daily functioning.

"The non-ADHD spouse may assume their ADHD partner is being passive aggressive when they are late, procrastinating, or forgetful," notes Dr. Goodman. "It may look like the ADHD partner is unmotivated to change or trying to annoy, when in fact the ADHD individual is impaired and unable to perform at the required level."

Most often the problematic behaviors of the ADHD partner are a function of an inability and impairment rather than a motivation issue. With this insight and understanding the non-ADHD spouse is often less frustrated.

If your spouse won't seek treatment, consider getting help for yourself. Meeting a trained mental health professional can help you develop a better understanding of your spouse's symptoms and assist you in developing the most effective ways to deal with those symptom.

Relationship Advice When Your Partner Has ADHD

You may find yourself wondering how you can cope with your ADHD partner and wondering how best to communicate and interact with your significant other. Some common concerns include:

• Feeling like your partner's parent

• Feeling like your partner is using an ADHD diagnosis as an excuse to behave worse

• Battling with your partner to take their medication regularly

• You've read up on ADHD to try to understand, but the reality of day-to-day life is difficult

• You feel like you're taking on all the responsibilities and it's wearing you down

- You need time to yourself but your partner is demanding 100% of your attention

- Your sex drives aren't matching up

- Feeling like a caregiver is taking away from the romance

- Your partner doesn't treat you with respect

- You cannot share secrets without them being broadcast

- Alleviating Your Concerns

If these concerns sound similar to yours, know that you are not alone in your frustrations. Many partners of ADHD adults do indeed experience the same problems described here. Understanding that the hyperactive, impulsive, emotional, and erratic responses are ADHD-related is good; that's the first step to improving the relationship. But using ADHD as an excuse is never helpful. If your partner continues to do this and casts off all responsibility for his or her behaviors and refuses to follow through with a treatment plan, things just won't get any better for you, your partner or your relationship.

If however, the two of you can sit down with his or her doctor and come up with a plan for addressing these behaviors, your relationship can thrive and the closeness you initially felt can return. It does take effort from both partners to make things better.

Avoiding the Parenting Trap

Many non-ADHD partners end up falling into the mothering role while their ADHD partner assumes the role of a child who has to be told what to do and needs someone to constantly take care of them. You both must try to step out of these roles. It is okay to assume responsibility for tasks your partner just isn't good at (for instance, maybe you are better at paying the bills and he is better at cooking meals), but make sure the jobs around the house are divided evenly so you don't wear yourself out.

Communication Is Critical

Open communication is key. The two of you must be able to address the problems without blame or accusations. Try to pick a time when you are both feeling relaxed and in a good mood. Then, in a matter-of-fact way make a list of concerns and a list of possible solutions. For example, you both have frustrations about your sexual relationship. You feel tired—probably pretty angry, too—and you don't feel romantic when you are "his mom" and constant caregiver and he is the child so much of the time. I imagine you don't feel romantic or respected either when you are grabbed or groped at other times. He likely feels rejected that you both have gone so long without sex. Medication may help his impulsive gropes, blurting out of your secrets, and overall hyperactivity. A regular date night may help bring back the romance.

Carving Out Time for Yourself

Talk with your partner about the importance of you having alone time. Without it, you will begin to feel resentment (if you don't already) toward him for denying you this time. He craves your attention. Address this by setting up regular one-on-one time where you can both focus on each other. Make a daily schedule where you plan in these times and stick to the plan. This way, you get to enjoy your alone time for a portion of the day, and he gets a regular time to receive your undivided attention during another part of the day.

Don't Forget to Laugh

Try to find the humor in things together. Forgive each other, but also move forward with you both making changes for the better in the relationship. Work with the doctor or couples counselor who is experienced and knowledgeable about the ways ADHD can affect relationships.

How Does ADHD Affect Sex Drive

There are many ways that attention deficit hyperactivity disorder (ADHD) can affect your sex life. If you live with ADHD, you might notice that you are hypersensitive to sensory stimulation, making sensual touch feel irritating and even annoying. Or perhaps your level of sexual desire changes drastically from one day to the next.

On the flip side, some people with ADHD have such a high sex drive and need for stimulation and novelty, such as pornography, that it causes problems in a partnership.

People with ADHD may also be prone to sexual risk-taking such as unprotected sex or having multiple sex partners. The disorder is associated with a drop in neurotransmitters, which may lead to these types of impulsive behaviors.

There's even something called post-orgasm irritability that can happen with ADHD, where the drop in dopamine following intense pleasure leads to feelings of sadness and depression.

If Your Partner Has ADHD

As the partner of someone living with this disorder, you might notice that your partner becomes distracted during intercourse and easily loses focus and interest, which you might interpret as rejection. It's important to understand that ADHD causes trouble concentrating in many areas of life, and sex is often no exception—and it usually has nothing to do with the person's interest in their partner.

Let's not forget the exaggerated feelings that someone with ADHD may experience, such as anger and frustration, can create feelings of conflict in any romantic relationship, and this conflict can result in difficulties connecting sexually as well.

How to Have a Better Sex Life With ADHD

First and foremost, it's crucial to take ADHD medications as prescribed, and the good news is, many of them don't lower sex drive or sexual desire. In fact, because they increase your ability to focus, they may actually improve your sex life. However, antidepressants are sometimes prescribed for ADHD, and they can indeed lower sex drive. If that is a significant issue or concern, bring it up with your physician. You may be able to lower the dose or switch medications.

Beyond that, there are several steps you can take to overcome your challenges from ADHD in the bedroom.

Communication is key. If your ADHD is causing sexual issues, tell your partner that your distraction or other ADHD-driven behaviors are not his or her fault and not a reflection of your level of desire and attraction. Share what you like and what bothers you during foreplay and sex. If you don't like certain smells or lighting, set up your environment in a way that is more comfortable for you. If you don't enjoy certain positions or types of sex, tell your partner what you prefer. If your partner has ADHD, encourage him or her to openly share with you and listen without judgment.

Get rid of distractions. Since it can be hard enough to stay engaged during intercourse, eliminate anything around you that might cause you to lose focus, such as the television. You might also practice releasing the stresses of the day through meditation, yoga, or journaling before getting under the sheets with your partner, to get ahead of any worries on your mind.

Seek the health of a qualified sex therapist or mental health professional. Many couples dealing with ADHD benefit from talk therapy and counseling to improve their sex lives. It helps open lines of communication and bring clarity to misunderstandings and arguments, leading to more intimacy and by extension, better sex.

20 Signs and Symptoms of ADHD in Girls

How the condition tends to present in females may surprise you

Attention deficit hyperactivity disorder (ADHD) has long been thought of as a condition affecting males (think an energetic boy who has trouble sitting still during class). However, more girls are being diagnosed as the understanding of how the condition can present differently depending on sex deepens. Girls are more likely to have inattentive ADHD, in which daydreaming and shyness are common, whereas it is more typical for boys to have hyperactive-impulsive ADHD or combined presentation.[1]

Living with undiagnosed ADHD can result in many disadvantages, such as a lack of accommodations in the classroom, low self-esteem, and self-blame. Gone undiagnosed, ADHD can even affect mental health well into adolescence and adulthood. Being aware of the different ways ADHD can present in your daughter can help you know when it might be time to see a doctor for an evaluation.

Common Characteristics

It is much easier to identify a child who is physically active and defiant as someone that would benefit from an ADHD evaluation than someone who seems distant or distracted. In girls, ADHD signs and symptoms tend to have these underlying commonalities:2

Compensates for Inattention

For many girls with ADHD, paying attention to the task at hand is their biggest challenge. They can get distracted by external events or drift off into a world of their own. For example, a bird outside a classroom window may take attention away from something more important in their environment, like a teacher announcing the date of an upcoming exam.

To compensate, a girl with ADHD may hyper focus on something she likes or is good at. She will put forth so much effort and concentration that parents or teachers may dismiss the possibility of ADHD. Sometimes this hyper focus is a coping strategy to keep herself entertained when something is boring. Other times, she may not feel she has any control over it.

Always in Motion

If a girl is hyperactive, she might be described as a "tomboy" because she likes physical activity and doesn't seem to enjoy the "typical things" a girl her age does. She might also be in motion in less obvious ways, perhaps doodling constantly or moving around in her chair.

Overly Sensitive and Has Problems With Impulse Control

A girl with impulsivity can be hyper-talkative and verbally impulsive, interrupting others, talking excessively, or changing topics again and again during conversations. She might blurt out words without thinking about their impact on others. Some girls are described as overemotional, "drama queens," and easily excitable.

ADHD symptoms can manifest very differently in each child. You may have a boy who has been diagnosed with ADHD, but never considered that your daughter who is having trouble in school might also have it too because her issues seem so different from his. ADHD symptoms in girls are often thought of as characters of a girl's personality rather than ADHD, which is why they are often overlooked or explained away.

Signs to Look Out For

Not all girls with ADHD will exhibit all of the following signs and symptoms.3 Conversely, having one or two of these does not equal an ADHD diagnosis in and of itself. However, if your daughter seems to exhibit a few of these symptoms on a continual basis, a discussion with an experienced professional may be beneficial.

- Difficulty maintaining focus; easily distracted

- Shifting focus from one activity to another

- Disorganized and messy (in her appearance and physical space)

- Forgetful

- Problems completing tasks

- Daydreaming and in a world of her own

- Takes time to process information and directions; seems like she doesn't hear you

- Looks to be making "careless" mistakes

- Often late (poor time management)

- Hyper-talkative (always has lots to say, but is not good at listening)

- Hyperreactivity (exaggerated emotional responses)

- Verbally impulsive; blurts out and interrupts others

- Seems to get easily upset

- Highly sensitive to noise, fabrics, and emotions

- Doesn't seem motivated

- Doesn't appear to be trying

- Seems shy

- Appears withdrawn

- Cries easily

- Might often slam her doors shut

- Seeking Help

If ADHD is diagnosed, it can be treated and managed. Interventions can be put in place, including behavior management techniques, organizational strategies, medication, counseling, and support.

Simply knowing she has ADHD can relieve a girl of a huge burden of guilt and shame. It can also free her from the damaging labels of being "spacey," "unmotivated," "stupid," or "lazy." She is none of those things; she simply has ADHD. Strategies can be put in place to make life a little easier and her future much brighter.

Myths About ADHD

Misconceptions and Myths About ADHD

Myth 1: ADHD Is Not a Real Disorder

ADHD is recognized as a disorder/disability by the Centers for Disease Control, the National Institutes of Health, the United States Congress, the Department of Education, the Office for Civil Rights, the American Medical Association, and every other major professional medical, psychiatric, psychological and educational association or organization. Part of the misunderstanding about ADHD stems from the fact that no specific test can definitively identify ADHD. A doctor cannot confirm the diagnosis through laboratory tests as they can other medical diseases such as diabetes. Though there is not yet a specific medical test for diagnosing ADHD, clear and specific criteria must be met for a diagnosis to be made. Using these criteria and an in-depth history and detailed information about behaviors, a reliable diagnosis can be made. An additional misconception may occur because symptoms of ADHD may not always seem clear-cut. We all experience problems with attention and focus to some degree.

For an individual with ADHD, however, these symptoms are so severe that they impair daily functioning. ADHD represents an extreme on a continuum of behaviors. Sometimes the behaviors are misunderstood. Symptoms of ADHD can certainly appear similar to other conditions. That is why the health professional making the diagnosis must first rule out any other pre-existing conditions or causes for the symptoms.

Myth 2: ADHD Is Caused by Poor Parenting

This myth has often created negative feelings of self blame in parents of children with ADHD. It is simply not true that poor parenting causes ADHD. What is true, however, is that positive parenting with clear and consistent expectations and consequences and a home environment with predictable routines can help manage symptoms of ADHD. Conversely, a home setting that is chaotic or parenting that is punitive and critical can worsen symptoms of ADHD.

Myth 3: Only Children Can Have ADHD

Though the symptoms of ADHD must be present by age 7 in order to meet the criteria for diagnosis, many individuals remain undiagnosed until adulthood. For some adults, a diagnosis is made after their own child is diagnosed. As the adult learns more and more about ADHD, he or she recognizes the ADHD traits in themselves. They may think back to their own childhood and recall the struggles in school and problems with attention that were never treated. It is often a huge relief to finally understand and put a name to the condition causing the problems. Thirty percent to 70 percent of children with ADHD continue to exhibit symptoms into adulthood. Often times, the hyperactive behaviors common with children decrease with age, but symptoms of restlessness, distractibility, and inattention continue. Left untreated adult ADHD can create chronic difficulties with work and in relationships and can result in secondary issues such as anxiety, depression and substance abuse.

Myth 4: You Have to Be Hyperactive to Have ADHD

This myth has lead to a lot of confusion about ADHD. Even the name of the condition itself Attention Deficit Hyperactivity Disorder — leads to misunderstanding. There are actually three different types of ADHD: the predominately hyperactive-impulsive type, the predominately inattentive type, and the combined type. The predominately inattentive type does not include symptoms of hyperactivity at all. Because of this, it is often referred to simply as ADD. An individual with the inattentive symptoms may present as daydreamy and easily distracted, disorganized, forgetful, careless. The predominately inattentive type of ADHD is much less disruptive to others around the individual. So it often gets overlooked, but it is no less stressful for the individual. It is also important to point out that adults with ADHD may lose some of the hyperactive behaviors that may have been present in childhood. Instead the hyperactivity is replaced with a sense of restlessness. Click on ADD verses ADHD to read more.

Myth 5: Use of Stimulant Medications Leads to Drug Abuse and Addictions

Research has actually found the opposite result. If left untreated, individuals with ADHD are at a higher risk of substance abuse. This is likely because secondary problems (such as anxiety or depression) develop from the untreated ADHD and the individual uses the illicit substances to help relieve the ADHD symptoms. It becomes a way of self medicating, though it is obviously not effective. For those who receive appropriate treatment, which often does include stimulant medications, the rate of substance abuse is much lower.

Myth 6: If You Can Keep Focused on Some Activities, You Do Not Have ADHD

It can be quite confusing to see someone with ADHD focus intently on an activity when ADHD seems to be an "attention deficit." It is actually more appropriate to describe ADHD as a condition in which individuals have difficulty regulating their attention. Though they may have extreme problems focusing, organizing, and completing certain mundane tasks, they are often able to focus intently on other activities that interest and engage them. This tendency to become absorbed in tasks that are stimulating and rewarding is called hyperfocus. Click on Hyperfocus and ADHD to learn more.

Myth 7: Medication Can Cure ADHD

Medications do not cure ADHD rather they help to control symptoms of ADHD on the day they are taken. ADHD is a chronic condition that does not go away, though symptoms may change or lessen over time. Many individuals develop coping and organizing strategies to help manage and control symptoms over their lifetime. Some individuals continue to need medical treatment through medications to help control their symptoms into adulthood.

ADHD and Your Sex Life

If you have attention deficit hyperactivity disorder (ADHD), it can cause problems with intimacy and lead to some communication problems.

How ADHD Can Affect Your Sex Life

You can have trouble paying attention during sex. Your mind might wander during foreplay, cuddling, or sex. That may seem normal to you, but your partner may see it as lack of interest.

Your mood or desires may change suddenly. One day you might like cuddling or a certain sex act. The next day, the same things might bother you.

Feelings like anger and loneliness may make you less interested in sex. They may also cause communication issues between you and your partner.

You may be drawn to risky behaviors, like unprotected sex. ADHD can lower levels of certain brain chemicals called neurotransmitters. That may make you more likely to take risks or be impulsive.

You may like to have different sex partners. This can make it harder to keep a long-term relationship and raise the chances of risky sex.

What You Can Do

Be open with your partner about your ADHD symptoms, such as trouble focusing and irritability. Reassure them it's not their fault.

Say what feels good for you. If you don't like being touched all the time, tell your partner when and how to touch you. This can prevent miscommunication and arguments.

Get rid of distractions. If you easily lose focus during sex, having sex in the dark may help you focus on the moment.

Take your medication as prescribed. Some ADHD drugs may boost your ability to focus and enjoy sex, while others can lead to a loss of sexual desire or ability. If that's the case, talk with your doctor and your partner about it.

Focus on intimacy, not sex. Trouble with focus can make it harder for you to get aroused or reach orgasm. Spend time on kissing, foreplay, and other acts besides intercourse. This can ease the pressure and help you and your partner enjoy yourselves.

Stay active. Regular exercise can help you focus and raise levels of feel-good brain chemicals such as dopamine. That can help you enjoy intimacy more, and may make you less likely to engage in risky sexual behaviors.

Consider talk therapy. Research shows that talk therapy can help ease ADHD symptoms that affect your sex life. A therapist can also help you better communicate with your partner in and out of bed.

Dating and Making Friends When You Have Adult ADHD

If you have ADHD, you might find it hard to date and to make friends. That's partly because good relationships require you to be aware of other people's thoughts and feelings. But ADHD can make it hard for you to pay attention or react the right way. That doesn't mean you can't find a romantic partner or good buddies. It just takes patience, self-awareness, and practical strategies.

How ADHD Makes Relationships Hard

The most common ADHD symptoms can complicate your social life.

Forgetfulness. Miss a friend's birthday bash? A no-show on your own date? You may well forget if you didn't write it down or set reminders.

Indifference. Many romances start intensely and cool down over time. But your ADHD brain can zap a crush too soon. Why? It's wired to shift attention from old to new more quickly. When your passion fades, it can leave your love interest confused or upset.

Life With Psoriasis: How to Stay Positive

Psoriasis doesn't have to rule your life. You can stay upbeat and comfortable in the skin you're in.

Social miscues. To connect with people, you need to be able to read body signals and social situations. ADHD can make you misunderstand other people's comments or not notice how they react to your behavior.

Miscommunication. You might not catch the emotional meaning behind words. You might easily overlook the sarcasm, fear, or other unspoken messages. That can lead to misunderstandings and hurt feelings.

Disorganization. Household clutter can drive a tidy roommate mad. But the tension can go higher if your ADHD leaves you overwhelmed or anxious at the thought of tackling the mess.

Sex and Intimacy. Your ADHD can get in the way of intimacy -- the emotional bond with your partner. Studies suggest that discomfort and fear of getting close may be stronger the more serious your symptoms are. At the same time, the impulsivity that's a common hallmark of ADHD can lead you to do risky things. People with the condition tend to start sex at a younger age, have more partners, and have unprotected sex more often.

What You Can Do

If you think your ADHD is coming between you and your friends or romantic interest, these tips may help make your relationships more mutually

Listen beyond words. Pay attention to body language and tone of voice, too. Get a trusted buddy to help you interpret conversations. She can help you pick up subtle social cues you might miss.

Watch others for clues on what to do, like where to sit or what to wear.

Role play with a friend or romantic interest to get feedback and improve social skills.

Talk face-to-face. Texts, emails, and phone calls can't give you important cues like tone of voice and eye contact you get from a direct conversation.

Concentrate. Look at the person's eyes and make a mental note not to interrupt. If your mind starts to wander, repeat what you hear in your head to stay focused.

Tell your partner. Some ADHD meds can cause sexual problems. Talk to your partner openly about this and any other issues that may affect your relationship.

Seek help. Therapy may give you insights and tools to manage relationships. Talk therapy, for example, could help you work through your frustrations and other emotions. Cognitive-behavioral therapy can teach you to recognize and change thoughts and behaviors that might be affecting your social life

ADULT ADHD & RELATIONSHIPS

Does your husband complain that you never listen? Does your wife say she feels like you're just one more child in the house? Have your friends lost patience with you because you're late all the time? ADHD could be to blame. The condition starts in childhood, but it can stay into adulthood. Some people don't even know they have ADHD until they're adults. And if you have it, it could be causing relationship problems.

5 Warning Signs

While everyone is different, some common problems seem to affect the relationships of adults with ADHD. Do the following complaints sound familiar to you?

1. "Do you even hear what I'm saying?"

If you have the condition, your loved ones and friends might have a hard time getting your full attention. That's one reason why they might get frustrated with you. On the other hand, you might feel like they're nagging you.

2. "You never pull your weight around here."

Mowing the lawn. Washing the dishes. Folding clothes. Household chores can be a challenge when you have adult ADHD. If the people you live with tell you that you aren't doing enough, take a step back and consider whether they're right. When was the last time you took out the trash? Is your clutter taking over the house? Your family members may be doing more than their fair share of keeping the household running smoothly.

3. "You never do what you say you're going to do."

You meant it when you said you'd get to your son's basketball game by 4:30 p.m. You really did. But then you got distracted at work, and your cell phone rang, and then you realized you needed to pick up the dry cleaning. And before you knew it, the game was over -- and you were in the dog house. "People with ADHD very much intend to do something when they say it. It's not like some problems where people lie or are deceitful," says Steven Safren, PhD, director of behavioral medicine in the department of psychiatry at Massachusetts General Hospital.

4. "How could you forget a-g-a-i-n?"

Do you feel like you're always getting blamed for forgetting things, when you know no one actually told you about them?

Consider this: The condition often causes people to forget things they're told. And that can lead to major problems in relationships. If people have been telling you for years that you're forgetful, it might be time to find out if they're right.

5. "I can't believe you bought that -- you know we can't afford it!"

Fights over finances tend to be another problem. A common ADHD symptom is doing things on impulse, and that includes buying things. Adults with the disorder can have reckless spending habits and trouble saving money.

What to Do

If you think you or someone you care about has adult ADHD, the first thing you should do is learn about the disorder and how it's diagnosed.

You can start by looking over free online resources from organizations like Children and Adults with Attention-Deficit/Hyperactivity Disorder (CHADD) and the National Center on ADHD. These sites can help you find local doctors, and support groups where you can meet people facing similar issues. You can also find out how to get tested for the condition.

Your Relationships

If you're diagnosed with the condition, work with your doctor to deal with the problems you're having day to day. Adult ADHD is often treated with a combo of medications, skills coaching, and psychotherapy, including couples counseling and cognitive behavioral therapy. If you have a spouse or partner, it's important for them to be involved. They often can tell which treatments are or aren't working. "It's a good scenario if someone does have a supportive partner, so they can work together in a positive way to address the disorder," Safren says. And the sooner you both work on repairing your relationship, the better.

Skills training or coaching can help people with adult ADHD come up with and reach relationship goals. This might include building skills that help you manage your time well and get organized.

As for how much improvement you can expect in your relationships, experts say each situation is unique. But "usually, couples can make their lives better and recapture some of the joy and romance that might have gone out of the relationship," says psychologist Arthur Robin, PhD, professor of psychiatry at Wayne State University in Detroit.

Sexual disorders are frequently found in adults with ADHD

Sexual dysfunctions and other sexual disorders are highly prevalent in adults with attention-deficit/hyperactivity disorder (ADHD), according to results of a recent study conducted at an outpatient adult ADHD clinic in the Netherlands. Researchers found that 39% of men and 43% of women with ADHD had symptoms of a sexual dysfunction, while 17% of men and 5% of women ADHD patients had symptoms of a sexual disorder.

Sex and ADHD

Symptoms of sexual disorders (such as sexual aversion) occur in about 40% of adults with ADHD. "Screening for sexual disorders should be therefore standard procedure during diagnostic assessment" of adults with ADHD, the authors wrote in an article in the journal ADHD Attention Deficit and Hyperactivity Disorders.

Previous research has suggested that impulsive behavior, exposure to risky situations, proximity to motivated offenders, and poorer guardianship may lead to decreased sexual health and well-being in adolescents and young adults with ADHD.

"We believe that symptoms of ADHD may lead to sexual disorders and sexual dissatisfaction," wrote senior researcher Denise Bijlenga, PhD, and colleagues from the PsyQ outpatient adult ADHD clinic in The Hague, Netherlands. "For example, continuous distractedness and inattentiveness may result in decreased sexual arousal and orgasmic problems."

Because sexual functioning hasn't been well studied in adults with ADHD, Dr. Bijlenga and colleagues sought to assess the prevalence of sexual dysfunctions and other sexual disorders in adults with ADHD by comparing these patients with members of the general population.

The researchers recruited 136 patients age 18 and older (76 men and 60 women) diagnosed at their ADHD clinic. The patients filled out two questionnaires that screened for sexual problems and sexual dysfunctions. For comparison, the researchers used two large studies on sexual health in the Netherlands for a representative sample of the Dutch population. After comparing the results, the researchers found:

The most prevalent dysfunctions in men with ADHD included orgasmic problems (14%), premature orgasm (13%), sexual aversion (13%), and negative emotions during or after sex (10%).

Compared with men in the general population, male ADHD patients more often reported sexual aversion (12% vs 1%) and little desire for sexual contact (6% vs

0%). However, hypersexuality was higher in the male ADHD group than in the general population (12% vs 5%). In general, men in the ADHD group were more sexually active but also less often satisfied with their sex life than men in the general population (27% vs 68%).

In women with ADHD, the most prevalent dysfunctions were sexual excitement problems (26%), orgasmic problems (22%), and sexual aversion (15%).

Compared with women in the general population, female ADHD patients more often reported sexual aversion (15% vs 4%) and sexual excitement problems (26% vs 3%), but were equally low in terms of hypersexuality (2% vs 2%). As with the male ADHD group, the female ADHD group was less often satisfied with their sex life compared with women in the general population (35% vs 65%).

Symptoms of inattention and impulsiveness may result in sexual problems for adults with ADHD, the researchers explained. "Sexual excitement problems may be associated with insufficient focus on sexual stimuli, caused by easily being distracted in ADHD," they noted.

"We also found that quite a few ADHD patients reported sexual aversion, and a lot of male patients also reported negative emotions during or after sex. These men and women do not feel safe and in control during sex," Dr. Bijlenga and colleagues wrote. "Sexual aversion may be the result of negative sexual experiences in the past and can be associated with low self-esteem, fear of intimacy, and insufficient relational skills, which are all more prevalent in ADHD patients. However, we do not know if this is also the case in our patient sample."

The researchers further investigated whether sexual dysfunction was associated with depression, anxiety, or a substance use disorder (or the use of stimulants or antidepressants) in any of the patients with ADHD. But they found that none of the associations were statistically significant.

One limitation of the study was that it was conducted among adult men and women treated in an outpatient ADHD clinic, and therefore can't be generalized to all adults with ADHD in the general population, the researchers noted. In addition, the ADHD patients in the study were younger than the respondents in the general population studies.

Nevertheless, further research—such as the etiological relationship between ADHD and sexual problems—should be investigated, Dr. Bijlenga and colleagues recommended. "Sexual arousal may temporarily increase dopaminergic function and diminish the severity of ADHD symptoms (like concentration difficulties, restlessness, difficulty to relax, or sleep). In this respect, it should be studied if sexual behavior is used as a coping strategy in ADHD."

ADHD and Relationships

The distractibility, disorganization, and impulsivity characteristic of adult Attention Deficit Hyperactivity Disorder (ADHD) can negatively impact multiple areas of life, but the symptoms associated with ADHD can be particularly troubling for relationships.

When one or both partners struggle with ADHD, intimate relationships can be damaged by misunderstandings, frustration, and resentment. The good news is that learning about how your ADHD affects the relationship can help you find strategies and tools to improve communication with your partner and develop a healthier, happier relationship as a result.

Understanding the Symptoms of Adult ADHD

The defining feature of ADHD is a persistent pattern or inattention and/or hyperactivity-impulsivity that interfere with functioning (in more than one area) for a period of at least six months. For adults, hyperactivity often manifests as restlessness or wearing others down.

- Failure to pay close attention to details

- Difficulty remembering information

- Difficulty following directions

- Difficulty concentrating or remaining on task

- Struggles to organize tasks

- Difficulty completing work on time

- Chronic lateness and forgetfulness

- Social intrusiveness – frequent interruptions or making important decisions without consulting others

- Hyper-focus: Intense focus on things of interest (i.e. shopping online, video games) or tasks that are rewarding/stimulating

- Reckless behavior

- Poor planning

- Easily stressed out

- Explosive temper

- Difficulty sitting still

- Excessive talking

- Easily bored

Symptoms of Adult ADHD that Interfere with Relationships

The biggest challenge to making the necessary changes to improve your relationship is to understand the symptoms that have the greatest impact on your partner. Once you know how your symptoms influence your behavior with your partner, you can learn how to manage them.

Adult ADHD can be tricky because symptoms vary from person-to-person. These specific symptoms can impact how you relate to your partner:

Inattention: Adults with ADHD can lose focus during conversations, which leaves the partner feeling devalued. Inattention can also lead to mindlessly agreeing to things that you later forget. This can be frustrating and lead to resentment.

Forgetfulness: Even when adults with ADHD are paying attention, they might still forget what was discussed.

This can cause others to see the person as unreliable or incapable.

Impulsivity: This symptom of adult ADHD can lead to frequent interruptions during conversations or blurting out thoughts without considering the feelings of others. This can result in hurt feelings.

Disorganization: Difficulty organizing and/or completing tasks can lead to household chaos. This can cause resentment and frustration for the partner, who might feel like he or she does more of the work at home.

Explosive temper: Many adults with ADHD have difficulty regulating their emotions. This can result in angry outbursts that leave partners feeling hurt or fearful.

While the adult with ADHD in the relationship is at risk of feeling micromanaged and overwhelmed with criticism, the non-ADHD partner might feel disconnected, lonely, or underappreciated. It's important to place the focus on how the ADHD symptoms impact the relationship, instead of blaming one another for a breakdown in the bond.

Work on Communication Skills

Communication often breaks down when one partner has ADHD. More often than not, the behaviors on the surface (i.e. she's always late for dinner) mask a deeper issue (he feels underappreciated because she never shows up on time.)

Couples also tend to fall into a "parent-child" dynamic, where the non-ADHD partner feels responsible for everything and the ADHD partner feels like a child. This chronic pattern of micromanaging and underachievement can result in feelings of shame and insecurity for the ADHD partner.

When couples work to improve communication skills, they can restore balance to the relationship. Try these strategies to communicate effectively with your partner:

Use "I feel" statements to focus on feelings and avoid blame

Communicate face-to-face as often as possible – nonverbal cues are important

Repeat and rephrase – to avoid allowing your mind to wander, repeat what your partner says and rephrase for clarification

Ask questions

Text yourself important takeaways from the conversation (especially if your partner asks you to assist with certain tasks)

Talk about how your symptoms impair your ability to remember things or follow through on tasks. Sharing your struggles helps your partner understand how ADHD impacts your behavior

Hold eye contact when listening

For long conversations, consider a fidget toy like a squeeze ball to keep your mind engaged

Focus on teamwork. To create balance in a relationship, two partners have to work together. Having ADHD doesn't mean that you can't find balance; it means that you have to rely on open and honest communication and feedback to find ways to help one another.

Divide tasks based on strengths. If ADHD interferes with your ability to pay bills on time or manage money, ask your partner to handle that task. When couples divide tasks based on their strengths, they get through their to-do lists without either partner feeling overburdened or resentful.

Evaluate the workload. Have a weekly meeting at a predetermined time to discuss the workload and rebalance the tasks if one of you is feeling overwhelmed. A weekly check-in gives you the chance to consider how you're doing with your household tasks and whether or not you need a change. Weekly check-ins are also a great opportunity to slow down and connect and plan time together to strengthen your bond. When one partner has ADHD, relationships can quickly become overwhelmed by the focus to attend to tasks together to reduce frustration, but it's just as important to spend time together enjoying each other's company.

Delegate tasks. You and your partner don't have to manage every aspect of the household independently (particularly if failure to complete tasks is a common problem impacting your relationship.) If you have children, assign age appropriate chores to help keep the house organized. Automatic bill pay can be very helpful for adults with ADHD. If you can afford it, you might also consider a monthly cleaning service.

Rely on routines. Routines, schedules, and visual planners (think wall-size whiteboard calendar) help adults with ADHD know what to expect, stay on task, and complete important tasks. When couples coping with ADHD use organizational systems to take some of the guesswork out of the daily grind, they can focus more on connection than completing tasks and chores.

10 Ways to Save Your Relationship

All you need is love, right? Wrong. If you or your partner has ADHD, follow these rules to foster communication, build trust, and reciprocate support.

Regardless of adult attention deficit disorder (ADHD or ADD), falling in love is easy. A rush of biochemical euphoria comes with "new love." Those of us with ADHD often hyper focus on romance, not just for the sake of romance, but also to increase those pleasure-producing neurotransmitters (dopamine) that are in short supply in our brains. Highly charged emotions are not part of lasting love. They are just feelings strong and wonderful feelings but you need much more to make an ADHD relationship last.

Relationships are hard, and when we accept that fact, we are dealing with reality, not the fantasy that "all you need is love." All we need is love? I don't think so. You need coping skills to compensate for your weaknesses and to save your relationship. What tools should you have in your relationship toolbox? Glad you asked.

ADHD Relationship Tool 1: Manage Symptoms

You and your partner must take ownership of your condition. Treat ADHD responsibly by using behavior therapy and/or appropriate medications to manage symptoms, increase dopamine, and help the brain work as it is supposed to. When you do all that, you should see a decrease in ADHD symptoms —like the inability to focus when your partner is talking to you or to follow through on tasks, such as paying bills on time.

Not being heard is a major complaint of those in intimate relationships with partners with ADHD. For many who have ADHD, listening to others is hard. To increase your listening skills, practice this exercise:

Sit down with your partner and let him talk for five minutes — or longer, if you can manage it. Make eye contact and lean toward him, even if you're not absorbing every word.

After five minutes of listening, summarize what you've heard. You might say, "Wow, it sounds like you had a really hectic day. The lousy commute, the awful meeting. At least you got to stop at the gym on the way home." After the exchange, do something you want to do. Say, "Now that you're home, would you mind watching Robbie while I go for a run?"

Your partner will probably be shocked, and pleased, that you have listened to him for a full five minutes.

Commit to Commitment

The main symptoms of ADHD — impulsiveness and the need for constant stimulation — can enhance, as well as threaten, relationships. Because adults with ADHD are impatient and easily bored, adventurous sexual activities are highly stimulating. Attraction to the new and different may make it difficult to stay monogamous. That's why it is vital to be committed to the idea of "relationship" — even more so than your partner.

I met a 93-year-old woman who had been married to the same man for more than 70 years. She told me that they had good times and bad times in their years together, and that she had never once considered divorce, though she joked that she had considered murder once or twice. She knew that she had to be more committed to the institution of marriage than to her husband to make the relationship work. There were times when the couple didn't feel committed to each other, but their dedication to their marriage got them through.

Use Laughter Therapy

Learn to laugh at yourself (not at your partner) and to take your problems a little more lightheartedly. ADHD causes us to do and say some pretty unusual things sometimes.

Rather than be wounded or angered by unintended words and actions, see them for what they are: the symptoms of a condition you're trying to manage. A good laugh allows you to move forward in the relationship. I know how difficult this can be. It is easy to be defensive because we have had to explain our behavior for years — when we acted impulsively or glossed over details due to lack of focus. Drop the defensiveness, then let go and move forward.

Forgive and Forget

It is tempting to point the finger at the other person and blame her for the problems in the relationship. But it takes two to tango. When we admit to the problems we may be causing, instead of dwelling on what our partner does wrong, we grow spiritually. When I acknowledge my own shortcomings — identify them, work on changing them, and forgive myself for not being perfect — it is easier to accept my partner and to forgive her shortcomings.

A phrase that sums up this forgive-and-forget concept is: "I did the best I could do in that moment. If I could have done better, I would have." This takes the sting out of a bad experience, and enables you and your spouse to talk with each other civilly. It is no longer about one of you "doing it again," it is about being human and making mistakes — something that is possible to forgive.

Seek Professional Help

Most married couples with one or more partners diagnosed with ADHD plan to be married "till death do us part." But as the realities of living together set in, little problems go unresolved and become bigger problems that seem insurmountable.

One of the common mistakes that troubled couples make is to wait too long before seeking professional help for their relationship. By the time they get to the therapist's office, they've already thrown in the towel, and are only looking for a way to validate their misery and justify their decision to divorce. Don't wait too long to get help. A licensed marriage and family therapist can teach communication and conflict resolution skills.

6 More ADHD Relationship Tools

Remember to keep doing the fun things you did together when you first fell in love.

Make a rule: Only one crazy person in the house at a time. If your partner is freaking out, you must stay cool and collected.

Go on a date every week.

Treat each other with respect. Learn to love each other's quirks.

Don't worry about who is right. The goal is to move forward — not to stay stuck in an argument. It is more important to have a mutually satisfying relationship than it is to be right all of the time.

Printed in Great Britain
by Amazon

86392006R00041